Chapter 1: Understanding Stress

What is Stress?

Definition:

Stress is your body's way of responding to any kind of demand or threat. When you perceive danger—whether it's real or imagined—your body's defenses kick into high gear in a rapid, automatic process known as the "fight-or-flight" response. This is your body's way of protecting you.

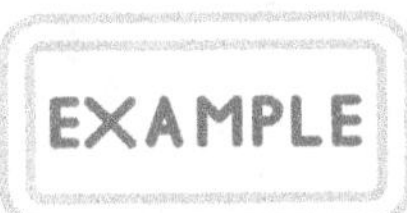

Imagine you're walking in a dark alley, and you hear footsteps behind you. Your heart races, and your muscles tense up. This is your body preparing to face danger or run away.

Positive Stress:

Not all stress is bad. Positive stress can motivate you to accomplish tasks and achieve goals. It can help you focus better and perform at your best.

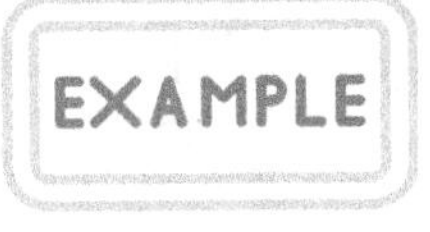

The nervousness you feel before giving a presentation can sharpen your focus and help you communicate more effectively.

Negative Stress:

Also called distress, this happens when stress feels overwhelming or unmanageable, leading to anxiety, frustration, or exhaustion.

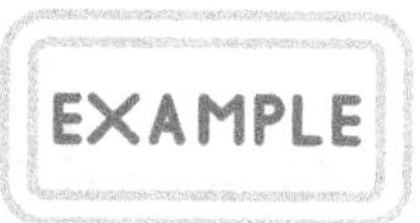

Chronic stress from constant work pressure without enough time to relax can lead to burnout, making you feel exhausted and overwhelmed.

Types of Stress:

Acute Stress:

This is short-term stress that goes away quickly. It's what happens when you need to slam on the brakes to avoid hitting a car, give a speech, or do something new and exciting. It helps you manage dangerous situations and makes you feel more alive and excited.

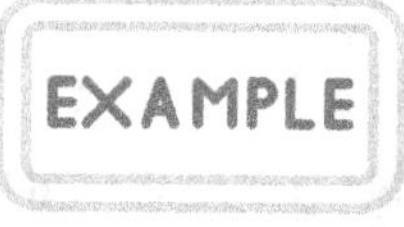

Feeling a rush of adrenaline when you're on a roller coaster or during a sports competition.

Chronic Stress:

This is stress that lasts for a longer period of time. You may have chronic stress if you are having money problems, an unhappy marriage, or trouble at work. When stress is constant, your body remains in a heightened state of alert, which can lead to health problems over time.

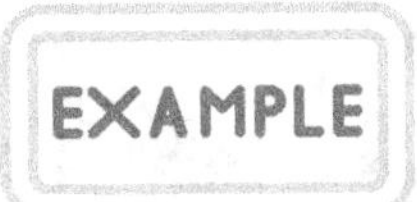

Worrying about paying bills every month or dealing with a difficult relationship can lead to ongoing stress.

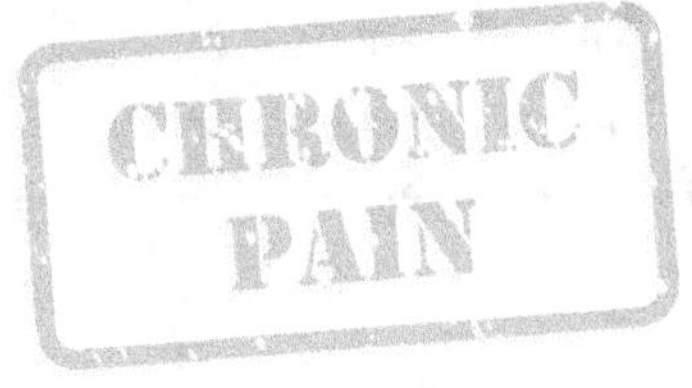

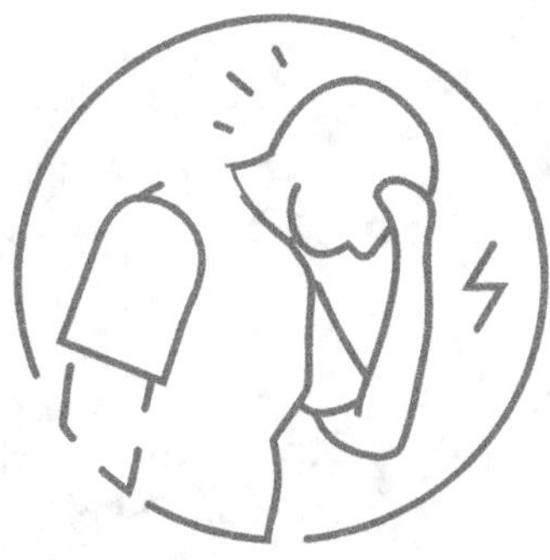

Physical Symptoms:

When you're stressed, your body reacts. Common symptoms include:

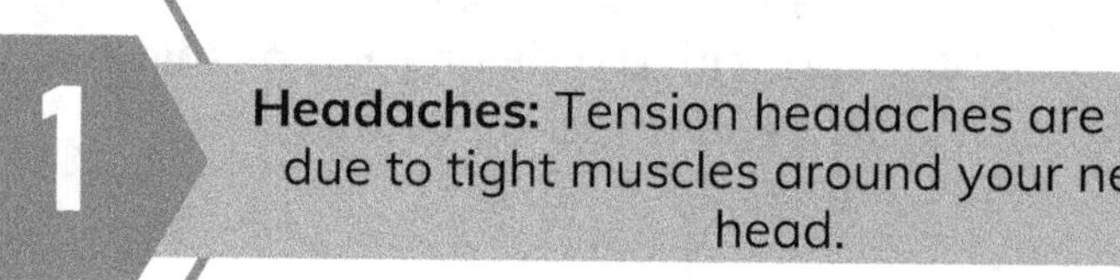

1. **Headaches:** Tension headaches are common due to tight muscles around your neck and head.

2. **Muscle Tension:** Stress causes your muscles to tighten, often leading to pain or discomfort, especially in your neck, shoulders, and back.

3. **Fatigue:** Chronic stress can drain your energy, leaving you feeling exhausted even after a full night's sleep.

4. **Stomach Issues:** Stress can disrupt your digestive system, causing nausea, indigestion, or stomach cramps.

Emotional Symptoms:

Feeling anxious, irritable, or sad are common emotional responses. Stress can also make you feel overwhelmed or unable to cope.

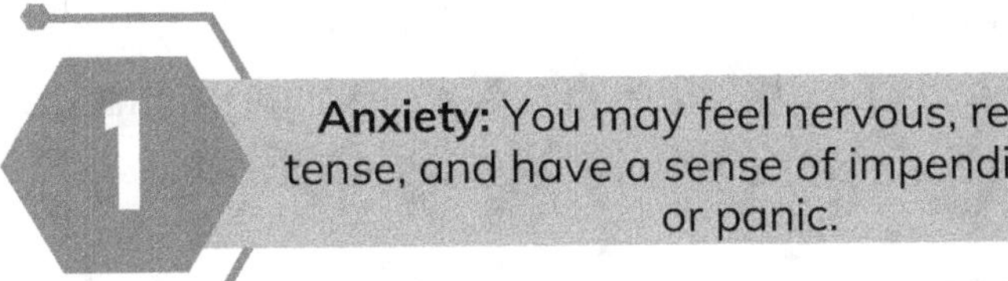

1 Anxiety: You may feel nervous, restless, or tense, and have a sense of impending danger or panic.

2 Irritability: Stress can make you more prone to angry outbursts or feeling frustrated over small things.

3 Sadness or Depression: Prolonged stress can lead to feelings of sadness, emptiness, or hopelessness.

4 Difficulty Concentrating: stress can make it hard to focus or remember things, leading to increased forgetfulness or confusion.

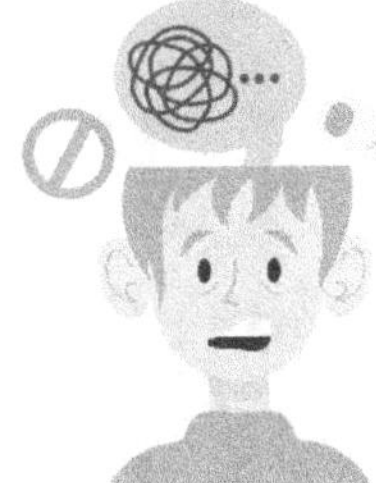

Chapter 2: Recognizing Your Stress Triggers

Common Triggers:

Work Pressure:

- <u>Deadlines:</u> Meeting tight deadlines or juggling multiple projects can increase stress levels significantly.

- <u>Long Hours:</u> Working overtime or not having enough time to relax can lead to burnout.

- <u>Conflict with Colleagues:</u> Disagreements or lack of support at work can make the environment more stressful.

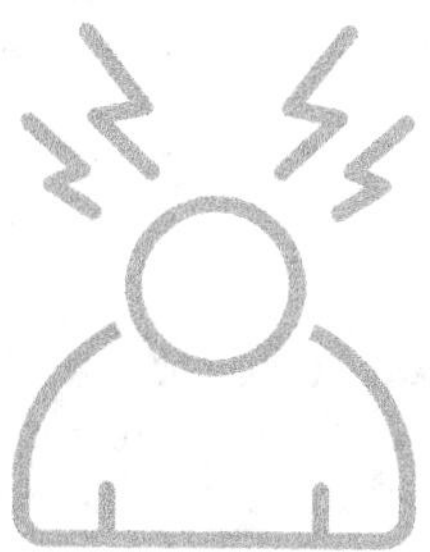

Family Issues:

Arguments, health concerns, or financial problems at home can be stressful.

- <u>Arguments or Conflicts:</u> Regular disagreements with family members can create a tense and stressful atmosphere.

- <u>Caring for Others:</u> Taking care of a sick relative or managing children's activities and school can add extra stress.

- <u>Relationship Problems:</u> Marital issues or conflicts with close family members can deeply affect your emotional well-being.

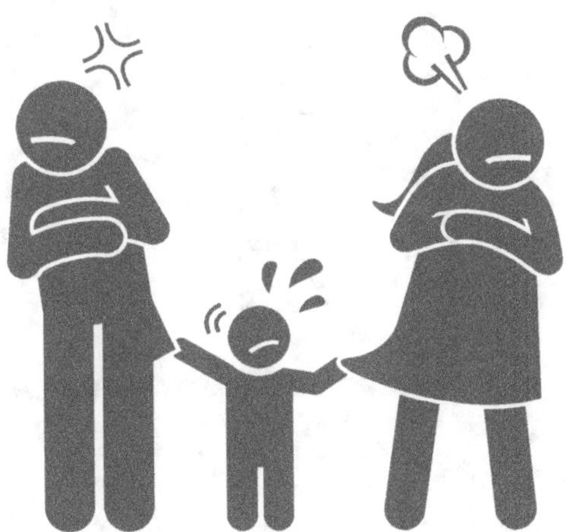

Financial Concerns:

Worrying about bills, debts, or unexpected expenses is a major source of stress for many people.

- <u>Debt:</u> Worrying about how to pay off loans or credit cards can cause ongoing anxiety.

- <u>Unexpected Expenses:</u> An unexpected medical bill or car repair can disrupt your financial stability, causing stress.

- <u>Job Insecurity:</u> Fear of losing your job or not being able to find work can keep you in a constant state of worry.

Keep a Stress Diary:

Write down when you feel stressed, what triggered it, and how you felt. This helps you spot patterns and understand what causes your stress.

- <u>What to Include:</u> Write down the date, time, and what you were doing when you felt stressed. Include what thoughts you had, how your body felt, and how you reacted (e.g., did you avoid a task or get irritable with someone?).

- <u>How It Helps:</u> Over time, you'll start to notice patterns in your stress. For example, you might realize that your stress peaks every Sunday evening because you're anxious about the workweek ahead.

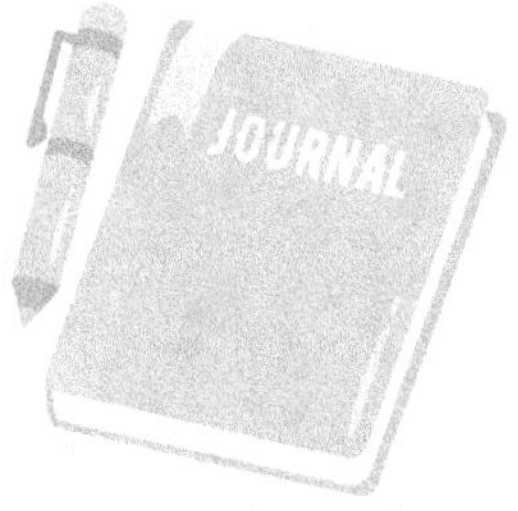

Note Patterns:

Do you always feel stressed on Monday mornings? Or maybe after certain meetings?
Noticing these patterns can help you find ways to manage stress better.

- <u>Identify Triggers:</u> Are there specific people, places, or situations that always make you feel stressed? Knowing these triggers can help you prepare or avoid them.

- <u>Track Responses:</u> Observe how you typically respond to stress. Do you reach for junk food, snap at loved ones, or withdraw from activities? Recognizing your responses is the first step to changing them.

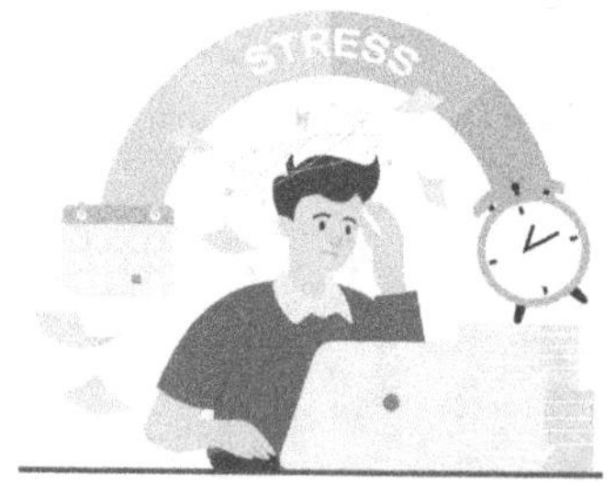

Chapter 3: Quick Stress Relief Techniques

Deep Breathing:

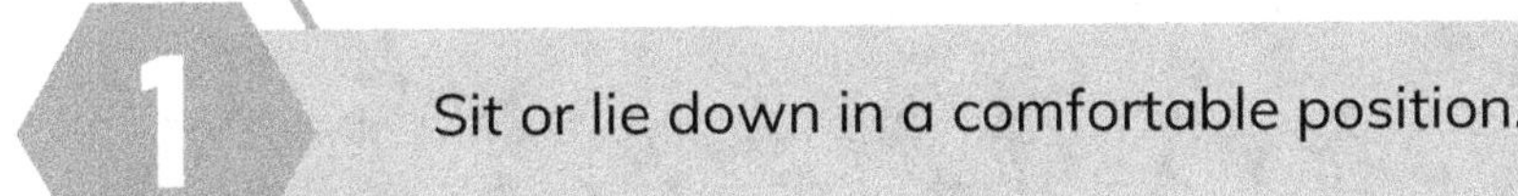

How to Do It:

1. Sit or lie down in a comfortable position.

2. Place one hand on your chest and the other on your belly.

3. Inhale deeply through your nose for 4 seconds, feeling your belly rise and hold your breath for 4 seconds.

4. Exhale slowly through your mouth for 6 seconds, feeling your belly fall and repeat it 5-10 times.

Why It Works:

Deep breathing sends a message to your brain to calm down and relax, reducing the "fight or flight" response.

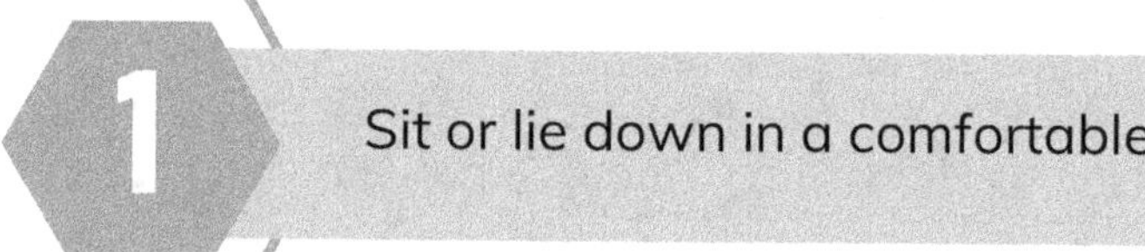

How to Do It:

1. Sit or lie down in a comfortable position.

2. Start with your toes. Tense the muscles for about 5 seconds, then release.

3. Move up to your calves, thighs, and so on, up to your neck and face.

4. Focus on the feeling of relaxation after releasing each muscle group.

Why It Works:

This technique helps release physical tension, making you feel more relaxed and calm.

How to Do It:

1 Close your eyes and take a few deep breaths.

2 Picture a peaceful scene in your mind, like a beach with waves gently crashing, a quiet forest with birds chirping, or a sunny meadow.

3 Engage all your senses—imagine the sounds, smells, and sensations you would experience in that place.

4 Stay in this scene for a few minutes, allowing yourself to fully relax.

Why It Works:

Visualization can distract your mind from stress and bring a sense of peace.

Chapter 4: Long-Term Stress Management Strategies

Exercise Regularly:

Why It Helps:

Physical activity boosts your mood by releasing endorphins (happy hormones). Even a brisk 20-minute walk can lower stress levels.

Tips to Start:

Find an activity you enjoy—dancing, yoga, or even gardening. Consistency is more important than intensity.

Healthy Diet:

Stress-Fighting Foods:

Omega 3	Rich Foods: Salmon, walnuts, and flaxseeds can help regulate stress hormones and improve mood.
Anti - oxidiant	Rich Foods: Berries, nuts, and dark chocolate combat oxidative stress in your body.
Carbo- hydrates	Complex Carbohydrates: Foods like oatmeal and whole-grain bread can boost serotonin, a brain chemical that helps you feel calm.

Avoid:

Too much caffeine, sugar, or processed foods can increase stress and anxiety.

Why It's Important:

During sleep, your body repairs itself and your mind processes the day's events. Not getting enough sleep can make stress and anxiety worse.

Tips for Better Sleep:

Create a Routine	Go to bed and wake up at the same time every day, even on weekends.
Limit Screen Time	Blue light from phones and computers can interfere with your sleep cycle. Try to avoid screens at least an hour before bed.
Relax Enviroment	Keep your bedroom cool, dark, and quiet. Consider using a white noise machine or blackout curtains.

Mindfulness Meditation:

How It Helps:

Mindfulness involves being present in the moment, which reduces stress and anxiety.
Meditation can help you focus, relax, and gain perspective.

Getting Started:

Start with 5 minutes of focusing on your breath each day. Gradually increase the time as you get comfortable.

Focus	Focus on your breath as it moves in and out of your body.
Breath	If your mind wanders, gently bring it back to your breath.
Body Scan	Close your eyes and mentally scan your body from head to toe, noticing any areas of tension and releasing them.

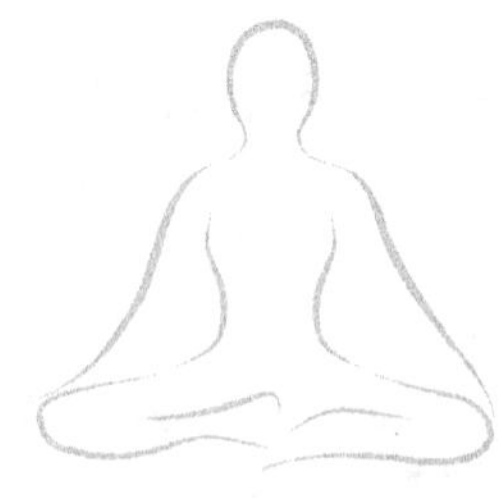

Chapter 5: Creating a Stress-Free Environment

Declutter Your Space:

Why It Matters:

A cluttered environment can lead to a cluttered mind, making it harder to focus and relax.
Keeping your space organized can help you feel more in control and less overwhelmed.

Quick Tips:

Choose one area, like your desk or a single drawer, to declutter. This prevents the task from feeling too overwhelming.

Donate or Discard: If you haven't used something in the past year, consider donating it or throwing it away.

Set a Daily Routine:
Spend 10-15 minutes each day tidying up.

Music:

Soft music or nature sounds can be incredibly calming. Try classical music, or sounds of the ocean or rainforest.

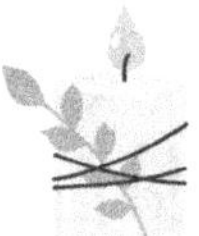

Scents:

Essential oils like lavender, chamomile, or sandalwood can promote relaxation. Use a diffuser, or put a few drops on your pillow.

Setting Boundaries:

Why It's Necessary:

Setting healthy boundaries is crucial to protect your time and energy.
It helps you avoid burnout and keeps your stress levels in check.

How to Do It:

Politely decline extra tasks that overwhelm you, and make sure to schedule time for self-care.

Chapter 6: Building a Support System

Talk to Someone:

Why It Helps:

Talking about your feelings with a trusted person can reduce stress by helping you process your thoughts and emotions. It can also provide new perspectives and solutions to your problems.

How to start:

Express Your Needs: You might say, "I'm going through a tough time and could use someone to talk to." It's okay to ask for help when you need it.

Choose the Right Person: Pick someone who is a good listener and supportive, whether it's a friend, family member, or coworker.

Be Honest and Open:
Share your feelings honestly, even if it's difficult.

When to Seek Help:

If stress is affecting your ability to function or enjoy life, it may be helpful to talk to a therapist.
They can provide techniques to manage stress and address underlying issues.

How It Works:

Therapists can teach you coping skills, help you understand your stress triggers, and support you through difficult times.

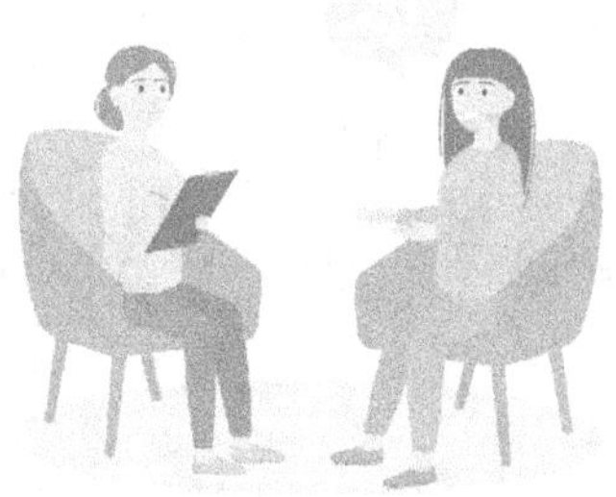

Why They're Beneficial:

Support groups offer a community of people who are going through similar experiences.
Sharing your story and hearing others can provide comfort and reduce feelings of isolation.

How to Find One:

Check local community centers, hospitals, or online forums for support groups related to stress, anxiety, or specific life challenges you're facing.

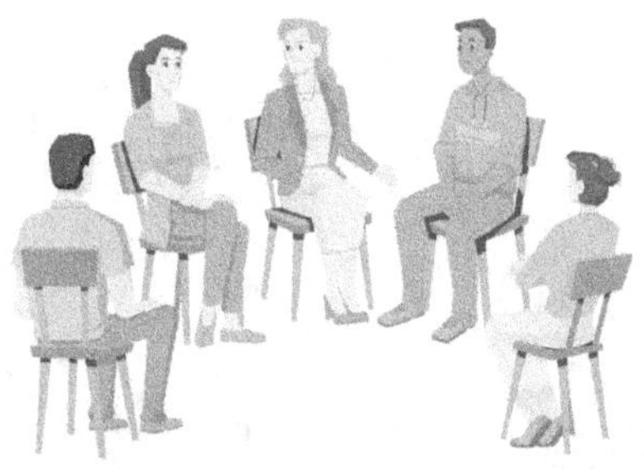

Chapter 7: Positive Lifestyle Habits

Gratitude Journaling:

How It Helps:

Focusing on what you're thankful for can shift your mindset from negative to positive. It's a powerful tool to boost your mood and reduce stress.

Getting Started:

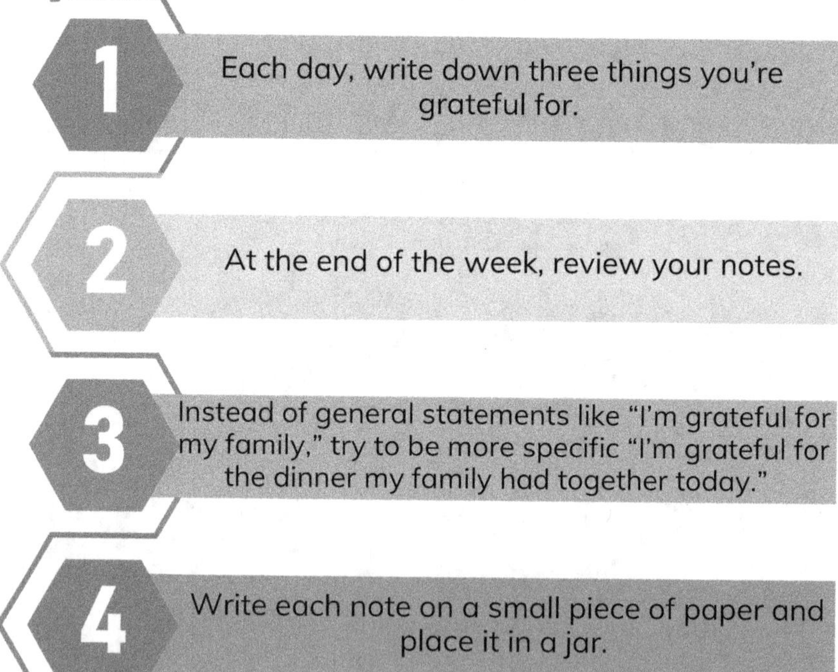

Hobbies and Creative Outlets:

Why They Matter:

Engaging in hobbies allows you to take a break from daily stresses and do something that makes you happy. It's a form of self-care that can improve your mental and emotional health.

Ideas to Try:

Cooking	Dancing	Swimming
Painting	Drawing	Photography
Knitting	Hiking	sining

Regular Breaks:

Why They're Important:

Taking breaks helps prevent burnout and maintains your productivity and focus throughout the day. It's essential for your mental and physical health.

Remember:

Stress is a normal part of life, but you don't have to let it control you.
By practicing the techniques in this eBook, you can take charge of your well-being.

Final Tips:

Be Kind to Yourself:

Don't be too hard on yourself if you have a stressful day or don't handle a situation as well as you'd like. Self-compassion is key to resilience.

Celebrate Small Wins:

Recognize and celebrate your efforts to manage stress. Each small step adds up and contributes to your overall well-being.

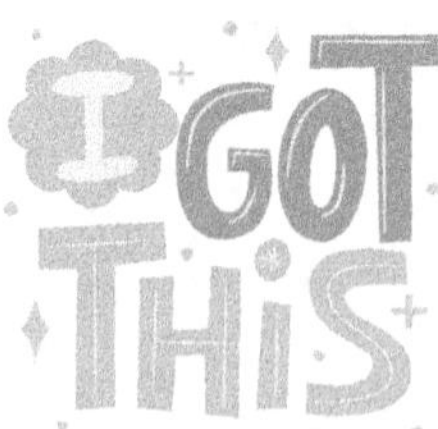